Empowered Bumps

The Ultimate Pregnancy Workout Guide for Strong and Healthy Moms-to-Be

Olivia Freedman

Table of content

INTRODUCTION

The Benefits of Exercise During Pregnancy

Exercise during pregnancy can have numerous benefits for both the mother and the baby. Here are some of the key benefits:

1. Improved Physical Health: Regular exercise can help improve cardiovascular health, strengthen muscles, and increase endurance. This can help the mother prepare for labor and delivery, which is a physically demanding process. Exercise can also help prevent or manage pregnancy-related conditions such as gestational diabetes, high blood pressure, and pre-eclampsia.

2. Reduced Risk of Excessive Weight Gain: Pregnancy often results in weight gain, but excessive weight gain can lead to health complications for both the mother and the baby. Exercise can help manage weight gain during pregnancy and reduce the risk of developing gestational diabetes or other pregnancy-related complications.

3. Improved Mood and Mental Health: Exercise has been shown to have a positive effect on mental health, including reducing stress and anxiety. This is especially important during pregnancy when hormonal changes can lead to mood swings and other emotional challenges.

4. Improved Sleep: Exercise can also help improve sleep quality, which is often disrupted during pregnancy due to physical discomfort, hormonal changes, and anxiety. Better sleep can lead to improved overall health and well-being for both the mother and the baby.

5. Improved Postpartum Recovery: Regular exercise during pregnancy can help improve postpartum recovery by strengthening muscles and increasing endurance. This can help the mother return to her pre-pregnancy fitness level more quickly.

It's important to note that pregnant women should always consult with their healthcare provider before starting or continuing an exercise program. They should also choose exercises that are safe and appropriate for their individual fitness level and stage of pregnancy. Overall, exercise during pregnancy can be a great way to stay healthy and prepare for the physical demands of labor and delivery.

Safety Guidelines and Precautions

When it comes to exercise during pregnancy, safety is of utmost importance. Here are some safety guidelines and precautions that pregnant women should keep in mind:

1. Consult with a Healthcare Provider: Before starting or continuing an exercise program during pregnancy, it's important to consult with a healthcare provider. They can provide guidance on safe exercises and help identify any conditions or complications that may require modifications to the exercise program.

2. Choose Low-Impact Exercises: High-impact exercises, such as running or jumping, can put excessive stress on the joints and increase the risk of injury.

Instead, pregnant women should choose low-impact exercises, such as walking, swimming, or prenatal yoga.

3. Avoid Overexertion: Pregnant women should avoid overexerting themselves during exercise. They should exercise at a moderate intensity level and avoid pushing themselves to exhaustion.

4. Stay Hydrated: Pregnant women should stay hydrated during exercise to prevent dehydration and overheating. They should drink water before, during, and after exercise.

5. Pay Attention to Warning Signs: Pregnant women should pay attention to warning signs during exercise, such as vaginal bleeding, abdominal pain, contractions, dizziness, or shortness of breath. If any of these symptoms occur, they should stop exercising immediately and consult with a healthcare provider.

6. Modify Exercises as Pregnancy Progresses: As pregnancy progresses, the body undergoes physical changes that may require modifications to the exercise

program. Pregnant women should modify exercises as needed to accommodate their changing bodies and avoid excessive strain or discomfort.

Overall, exercise during pregnancy can be safe and beneficial with proper precautions and guidance. Pregnant women should prioritize safety and listen to their bodies to ensure a healthy and successful pregnancy.

CHAPTER 1

Getting Started

Assessing Your Fitness Level

Assessing your fitness level is an important first step in developing a safe and effective exercise program during pregnancy. Here are some key factors to consider when assessing your fitness level:

1. Pre-Pregnancy Fitness Level: Your pre-pregnancy fitness level can provide a good starting point for assessing your current fitness level. If you were physically active before becoming pregnant, you may be able to continue with some of the same exercises, with modifications as needed.

2. Current Physical Activity Level: It's important to take into account your current physical activity level when assessing your fitness level during pregnancy. If you have been sedentary for a period of time, you may

need to start with light exercises and gradually increase intensity as your body adapts.

3. Physical Changes During Pregnancy: Pregnancy can cause physical changes that may affect your fitness levels, such as weight gain, changes in balance, and decreased flexibility. It's important to take these changes into account when assessing your fitness level and choosing appropriate exercises.

4. Health Conditions or Complications: If you have any health conditions or complications during pregnancy, such as gestational diabetes or high blood pressure, these can affect your fitness level and may require modifications to your exercise program.

5. Availability of Equipment or Facilities: When assessing your fitness level, consider what equipment or facilities are available to you for exercise. For example, if you have access to a pool, swimming may be a good exercise option, while if you do not have access to a gym, bodyweight exercises may be a better choice.

Overall, assessing your fitness level during pregnancy is an important step in developing a safe and effective exercise program. Be sure to take into account your pre-pregnancy fitness level, current physical activity level, physical changes during pregnancy, any health conditions or complications, and the availability of equipment or facilities. Consult with your healthcare provider for guidance on choosing safe and appropriate exercises.

Setting Realistic Goals

Setting realistic goals is an important aspect of developing a successful exercise program during pregnancy. Here are some key factors to consider when setting goals:

1. Pregnancy-Specific Goals: When setting goals during pregnancy, it's important to keep in mind the unique physical and emotional changes that occur during this time. Examples of pregnancy-specific goals may include preparing for labor and delivery, managing weight gain, or reducing stress.

2. Personal Goals: It's important to consider your personal goals when setting exercise goals during pregnancy. These goals may be related to improving cardiovascular health, building strength and endurance, or maintaining a healthy lifestyle.

3. Fitness Level and Physical Ability: When setting goals, it's important to take into account your current fitness level and physical ability. Setting overly ambitious goals that are not achievable can lead to frustration and disappointment, as well as increase the risk of injury.

4. Time and Availability: Consider your time constraints and availability when setting exercise goals. It may be unrealistic to set a goal of exercising for an hour every day if you have a busy schedule or other responsibilities to attend to.

5. Monitoring Progress: Setting goals is only the first step. It's important to monitor your progress and adjust your goals as needed. This can help keep you motivated and on track to achieving your goals.

Overall, setting realistic goals is an important aspect of developing a successful exercise program during pregnancy. Consider pregnancy-specific goals, personal goals, fitness level and physical ability, time and availability, and monitor progress when setting goals. Consult with your healthcare provider for guidance on setting safe and appropriate goals.

Choosing the Right Workout Program

Choosing the right workout program is essential for achieving your fitness goals during pregnancy. Here are some key factors to consider when choosing a workout program:

1. Safety: Safety should always be the top priority when choosing a workout program during pregnancy. Look for programs that are specifically designed for pregnant women, or consult with a healthcare provider to ensure that the program you choose is safe and appropriate.

2. Variety: A good workout program should include a variety of exercises to target different muscle groups

and prevent boredom. Look for programs that incorporate a mix of cardio, strength training, and stretching exercises.

3. Intensity: The intensity of the workout program should be appropriate for your fitness level and physical ability. Be sure to choose a program that is challenging but not overly strenuous, and that can be modified as needed throughout your pregnancy.

4. Duration: Consider the duration of the workout program when choosing a program. Programs that are too long or too short may not be practical for your schedule or fitness level.

5. Accessibility: Look for a workout program that is accessible and convenient for you. This may include programs that can be done at home or in a gym, and that do not require a lot of specialized equipment.

6. Support: Choosing a workout program that includes support and guidance can help keep you motivated and on track. Look for programs that include a community

or support group, or that provide guidance from a certified fitness professional.

Overall, choosing the right workout program is an important aspect of developing a successful exercise program during pregnancy. Consider safety, variety, intensity, duration, accessibility, and support when choosing a program, and consult with a healthcare provider for guidance on choosing safe and appropriate exercises.

CHAPTER 2

Prenatal Yoga

Benefits of Prenatal Yoga

Prenatal yoga is a popular form of exercise for pregnant women that offers a range of physical and mental benefits. Here are some of the benefits of prenatal yoga:

1. Reduces stress and anxiety: Pregnancy can be a stressful time, and prenatal yoga can help reduce stress and anxiety. The breathing techniques and meditation practiced in yoga can help calm the mind and reduce tension in the body.

2. Improves flexibility and balance: As pregnancy progresses, the body undergoes many changes that can affect flexibility and balance. Prenatal yoga can help improve flexibility and balance, which can reduce the risk of falls and improve overall comfort during pregnancy.

3. Strengthens muscles: Prenatal yoga includes a variety of poses that can help strengthen muscles, particularly in the hips, pelvis, and back. Strengthening these muscles can help prepare the body for labor and delivery, as well as reduce the risk of back pain and other discomforts during pregnancy.

4. Improves circulation: The breathing techniques practiced in prenatal yoga can help improve circulation, which can reduce swelling and other symptoms associated with pregnancy.

5. Enhances relaxation and sleep: Prenatal yoga can help promote relaxation and improve sleep quality, which is important for overall health and well-being during pregnancy.

6. Promotes bonding with baby: Prenatal yoga classes often include exercises and meditation that promote bonding with the growing baby. This can help expectant mothers feel more connected to their babies and enhance the overall pregnancy experience.

Overall, prenatal yoga is a safe and effective form of exercise for pregnant women that offers a range of physical and mental benefits. Consult with a healthcare provider and a certified prenatal yoga instructor to develop a safe and effective yoga practice during pregnancy.

Basic Poses and Modifications

Prenatal yoga is a safe and effective form of exercise for pregnant women, and there are many basic yoga poses that can be adapted or modified for the pregnant body. Here are some of the basic prenatal yoga poses and modifications:

1. Mountain Pose: Stand with your feet hip-width apart, grounding down through your feet. As you inhale, raise your arms overhead, keeping your shoulders relaxed. Modifications may include standing with your back against a wall or using a chair for support.

2. Cat-Cow Pose: Begin on your hands and knees, with your wrists directly under your shoulders and your

knees directly under your hips. As you inhale, arch your back and lift your head and tailbone. As you exhale, round your spine and bring your chin to your chest.

3. Downward-Facing Dog: Start on your hands and knees, with your hands shoulder-width apart and your knees hip-width apart. As you exhale, lift your hips and straighten your arms and legs. Modifications may include using a chair for support or practicing a modified downward-facing dog with your knees bent.

4. Warrior I Pose: Step your left foot back, keeping your left heel lifted. Bend your right knee and lift your arms overhead. Keep your hips facing forward and hold for several breaths. Repeat on the other side.

5. Triangle Pose: From Warrior I, straighten your right leg and extend your arms out to the sides. As you exhale, hinge at the hip and reach your right hand toward your right foot. Keep your left hand lifted and your gaze forward. Modifications may include using a chair for support or practicing with your hand on your hip instead of reaching for your foot.

6. Child's Pose: Begin on your hands and knees, then bring your hips back toward your heels and stretch your arms forward. Rest your forehead on the ground and take several deep breaths.

It's important to listen to your body during prenatal yoga and modify poses as needed. Avoid any poses that feel uncomfortable or cause pain, and be sure to consult with a certified prenatal yoga instructor for guidance on safe modifications. With regular practice, prenatal yoga can help promote strength, flexibility, relaxation, and overall well-being during pregnancy.

Sequencing and Breathing Techniques

Sequencing and breathing techniques are essential components of a safe and effective prenatal yoga practice. Here are some tips for sequencing and breathing in prenatal yoga:

1. Sequencing: When sequencing a prenatal yoga practice, it's important to start with gentle warm-up poses and gradually build up to more challenging poses.

Be sure to include poses that focus on strengthening the muscles needed for labor and delivery, such as the pelvic floor and the muscles of the back and legs. End the practice with restorative poses and a final relaxation pose.

2. Breathing techniques: Deep breathing and relaxation techniques can be especially helpful during pregnancy and labor. In prenatal yoga, the focus is on breathing into the belly rather than the chest, which can help calm the nervous system and reduce stress. Techniques such as Ujjayi breath (ocean-sounding breath) and Nadi Shodhana (alternate nostril breathing) can be especially beneficial during pregnancy.

3. Modifying poses for breathing: When practicing yoga poses, it's important to maintain deep and even breaths. This may require modifying certain poses, such as using props or modifying the pose to allow for deeper breathing. For example, in a forward bend, it may be helpful to bend the knees slightly and use a prop to support the head, allowing for deeper breathing.

4. Incorporating meditation: Meditation can be a powerful tool for reducing stress and promoting relaxation during pregnancy. Incorporate simple meditation techniques, such as focusing on the breath or repeating a mantra, into your prenatal yoga practice.

Overall, sequencing and breathing techniques are important components of a safe and effective prenatal yoga practice. Consult with a certified prenatal yoga instructor for guidance on sequencing and breathing techniques that are safe and appropriate for your pregnancy. With regular practice, prenatal yoga can help promote physical strength, flexibility, and relaxation during pregnancy.

CHAPTER 3

Strength Training

Benefits of Strength Training

Strength training is a type of exercise that involves using resistance to build muscle strength and endurance. While it may seem counterintuitive to engage in strength training during pregnancy, there are actually many benefits to this type of exercise.

1. Builds overall strength: As your body changes during pregnancy, it's important to maintain overall strength and muscle tone. Strength training can help prevent muscle imbalances, improve posture, and reduce the risk of injury.

2. Supports a healthy pregnancy: Strength training can help improve overall health and reduce the risk of pregnancy-related complications, such as gestational diabetes and preeclampsia. It can also help prepare the body for the physical demands of labor and delivery.

3. Supports postpartum recovery: Strength training during pregnancy can help support postpartum recovery by maintaining muscle strength and endurance. This can help you bounce back more quickly after delivery and may reduce the risk of postpartum complications.

4. Boosts mood and energy: Exercise, including strength training, can help boost mood and energy levels during pregnancy. This can help reduce stress and improve overall well-being.

5. Improves bone density: Strength training can help improve bone density, which is especially important during pregnancy when calcium demands increase. This can help reduce the risk of osteoporosis later in life.

It's important to work with a certified personal trainer or prenatal fitness specialist to develop a safe and effective strength training program during pregnancy. This may include modifications to certain exercises and avoiding exercises that may be unsafe during pregnancy, such as those that require lying on the back or involving high-impact movements. With proper guidance, strength training can be a safe and effective form of exercise during pregnancy.

Basic Exercises and Modifications

When it comes to strength training during pregnancy, there are a variety of exercises that can be modified to ensure safety and effectiveness. Here are some basic exercises and modifications that may be included in a prenatal strength training program:

1. Squats: Squats are a great exercise for building leg strength and preparing the body for labor. To modify squats during pregnancy, it may be helpful to use a chair or wall for support and to avoid deep squats that may strain the pelvic floor.

2. Lunges: Lunges are another effective exercise for building leg strength. To modify lunges during pregnancy, it may be helpful to use a chair or wall for

support and to avoid deep lunges that may cause instability or discomfort.

3. Push-ups: Push-ups are a great exercise for building upper body strength. To modify push-ups during pregnancy, it may be helpful to perform them on an incline (using a wall or bench for support) or to perform a modified push-up on the knees.

4. Rows: Rows are an effective exercise for building back strength. To modify rows during pregnancy, it may be helpful to use lighter weights and avoid exercises that require lying on the stomach.

5. Pelvic tilts: Pelvic tilts are a gentle exercise that can help improve pelvic stability and reduce lower back pain during pregnancy. To perform a pelvic tilt, lie on your back with your knees bent and feet flat on the floor. Inhale to prepare, then exhale as you tilt your pelvis upward, pressing your lower back into the floor. Hold for a few seconds, then release and repeat.

It's important to work with a certified personal trainer or prenatal fitness specialist to develop a strength training program that is safe and effective for your individual needs and fitness level. Modifications may need to be made throughout pregnancy as the body changes and adapts. By incorporating basic exercises and modifications, strength training can be a safe and effective form of exercise during pregnancy.

Progression and Overload

In strength training, progression, and overload are key principles that are used to continually challenge the body and improve fitness levels. During pregnancy, it's important to approach these principles with caution and to work closely with a certified personal trainer or prenatal fitness specialist to ensure safety and effectiveness.

Progression refers to the gradual increase in difficulty or intensity of an exercise over time. This can be achieved in a variety of ways, such as increasing the weight lifted, performing more repetitions or sets, or increasing the difficulty of the exercise itself. When progressing an exercise during pregnancy, it's important to take into account the changes that are occurring in the body and to progress at a pace that is appropriate for your individual needs and fitness level.

Overload refers to the stress placed on the body during exercise that causes adaptation and improvement. This stress must be progressively increased over time to continue to challenge the body and promote improvement. However, during pregnancy, it's important to approach overload with caution and to avoid overexertion or excessive stress on the body.

To incorporate progression and overload into a prenatal strength training program, it may be helpful to start with basic exercises and gradually increase the difficulty or intensity over time. It's important to listen to your body and to modify exercises as needed to ensure safety and avoid overexertion. As the body changes during pregnancy, modifications may need to be made to ensure safety and effectiveness.

Working with a certified personal trainer or prenatal fitness specialist can be helpful in developing a safe and effective strength training program that incorporates principles of progression and overload in a way that is appropriate for your individual needs and fitness level. By approaching these principles with caution and incorporating modifications as needed, strength training can be a safe and effective form of exercise during pregnancy.

CHAPTER 4

Cardiovascular Exercise

Benefits of Cardiovascular Exercise

Cardiovascular exercise, also known as cardio or aerobic exercise, is any form of physical activity that elevates the heart rate and increases oxygen consumption. During pregnancy, cardiovascular exercise can provide a variety of benefits for both the mother and the developing baby.

1. Improved cardiovascular health: Cardiovascular exercise can improve heart health by strengthening the heart muscle and improving blood flow throughout the body. This can help reduce the risk of heart disease and other cardiovascular conditions.

2. Increased energy and endurance: Regular cardiovascular exercise can increase energy levels and improve endurance, making it easier to perform daily activities and maintain overall fitness levels.

3. Reduced risk of gestational diabetes: Studies have shown that regular cardiovascular exercise can help reduce the risk of developing gestational diabetes, a condition that affects some women during pregnancy.

4. Improved mood and mental health: Cardiovascular exercise has been shown to improve mood and reduce symptoms of depression and anxiety. This can be especially beneficial during pregnancy when hormonal changes can contribute to mood swings and other emotional challenges.

5. Better sleep: Regular cardiovascular exercise can improve sleep quality and reduce the incidence of sleep disturbances, which are common during pregnancy.

6. Reduced risk of preterm labor: Some studies have suggested that regular cardiovascular exercise may help reduce the risk of preterm labor, although more research is needed in this area.

Some examples of safe cardiovascular exercises during pregnancy include brisk walking, swimming, cycling, and low-impact aerobics. It's important to work with a certified personal trainer or prenatal fitness specialist to develop a safe and effective cardiovascular exercise program that is appropriate for your individual needs and fitness level. By incorporating cardiovascular exercise into a prenatal fitness program, mothers-to-be can enjoy a variety of health benefits for themselves and their developing babies.

Safe and Effective Activities

When it comes to safe and effective activities during pregnancy, it's important to choose activities that are low-impact, non-jarring, and that don't involve contact sports or other activities that carry a high risk of injury. Here are some examples of safe and effective activities for pregnant women:

1. Walking: Walking is a low-impact exercise that can be done indoors or outdoors, and it doesn't require any special equipment. It's a great way to improve

cardiovascular fitness and maintain overall health during pregnancy.

2. Swimming: Swimming is another low-impact exercise that can be a great way to stay active during pregnancy. It provides a full-body workout and can help relieve pressure on the joints and muscles.

3. Prenatal yoga: Prenatal yoga is a gentle form of exercise that can help improve flexibility, balance, and strength. It also incorporates breathing and relaxation techniques that can help reduce stress and anxiety.

4. Pilates: Pilates is a low-impact exercise that focuses on strengthening the core muscles and improving posture. It can be a great way to maintain strength and flexibility during pregnancy.

5. Stationary cycling: Stationary cycling is a low-impact exercise that provides a great cardiovascular workout without putting pressure on the joints. It's also a good option for women who prefer indoor exercise.

6. Strength training: Strength training can be a safe and effective form of exercise during pregnancy, as long as it's done with proper technique and under the guidance of a certified personal trainer or prenatal fitness specialist. Exercises that focus on the major muscle groups, such as squats, lunges, and rows, can help maintain strength and muscle tone.

It's important to remember that every pregnancy is different, and what may be safe and effective for one woman may not be appropriate for another. It's important to consult with a healthcare provider and work with a certified personal trainer or prenatal fitness specialist to develop a safe and effective exercise program that is appropriate for your individual needs and fitness level.

Monitoring Intensity and Heart Rate

During pregnancy, it's important to monitor exercise intensity and heart rate to ensure that the exercise program is safe and effective. Here are some tips for monitoring exercise intensity and heart rate during pregnancy:

1. Use the Rate of Perceived Exertion (RPE): The RPE is a subjective measure of how hard you feel like you're working during exercise. On a scale of 1 to 10, with 1 being very light activity and 10 being maximum effort, you should aim to keep your RPE between 5 and 7 during pregnancy.

2. Use a Heart Rate Monitor: A heart rate monitor can be a helpful tool for monitoring exercise intensity during pregnancy. Aim to keep your heart rate below 140 beats per minute (BPM) during exercise, although some healthcare providers may recommend a lower maximum heart rate.

3. Avoid Overexertion: Avoid pushing yourself too hard during exercise, as this can increase the risk of injury and complications during pregnancy. If you feel fatigued, short of breath, or dizzy, stop exercising immediately and rest.

4. Modify Your Exercise Program: As your pregnancy progresses, you may need to modify your exercise

program to accommodate changes in your body. This may include reducing the intensity or duration of your workouts or switching to lower-impact activities.

5. Consult with Your Healthcare Provider: It's important to consult with your healthcare provider before starting any exercise program during pregnancy. Your healthcare provider can help you determine what exercise program is safe and effective for you based on your individual needs and health status.

By monitoring exercise intensity and heart rate during pregnancy, you can ensure that your exercise program is safe and effective and that you're getting the most out of your workouts without putting yourself or your baby at risk.

CHAPTER 5

Pelvic Floor Exercises

The Importance of Pelvic Floor Health

During pregnancy, the pelvic floor muscles undergo significant changes and can become weakened or stretched. These muscles play an important role in supporting the uterus, bladder, and rectum, and maintaining bowel and bladder control. Pelvic floor health is important for overall health and well-being during pregnancy and postpartum. Here are some reasons why pelvic floor health is so important:

1. Preventing Incontinence: Weak pelvic floor muscles can lead to incontinence, or the loss of bladder or bowel control. This can be particularly common during pregnancy and postpartum. By strengthening the pelvic floor muscles, you can help prevent incontinence and maintain bladder and bowel control.

2. Preparing for Labor and Delivery: The pelvic floor muscles play an important role in supporting the uterus and helping to push the baby out during delivery. By strengthening these muscles during pregnancy, you can prepare your body for labor and delivery and potentially reduce the risk of complications during childbirth.

3. Supporting Recovery Postpartum: After childbirth, the pelvic floor muscles may be weakened or stretched, which can lead to discomfort and complications such as incontinence or pelvic organ prolapse. By maintaining good pelvic floor health during pregnancy and postpartum, you can support your recovery and reduce the risk of complications.

4. Improving Sexual Health: The pelvic floor muscles are also important for sexual health and function. Strong pelvic floor muscles can help improve sensation and reduce the risk of sexual dysfunction.

To maintain good pelvic floor health during pregnancy, it's important to practice pelvic floor exercises, also known as Kegels. These exercises involve contracting and relaxing the pelvic floor muscles and can be done anywhere, anytime. It's also important to avoid activities that can put unnecessary strain on the pelvic floor, such as heavy lifting or high-impact exercise. By prioritizing pelvic floor health during pregnancy, you can improve your overall health and well-being, and potentially reduce the risk of complications during and after childbirth.

Kegels and Other Pelvic Floor Exercises

Kegels are a type of pelvic floor exercise that involve contracting and relaxing the muscles of the pelvic floor. These exercises can be done during pregnancy and postpartum to help maintain good pelvic floor health and prevent complications such as incontinence or pelvic organ prolapse. Here's how to do Kegels:

1. Identify the Pelvic Floor Muscles: To do Kegels, it's important to first identify the pelvic floor muscles. You can do this by stopping the flow of urine midstream. The muscles that you use to do this are the pelvic floor muscles.

2. Contract the Muscles: Once you've identified the pelvic floor muscles, contract them by squeezing them as if you're trying to stop the flow of urine. Hold the contraction for 5 seconds, then release.

3. Relax the Muscles: After holding the contraction for 5 seconds, relax the muscles for 5 seconds before starting the next contraction.

4. Repeat: Repeat this cycle of contraction and relaxation for 10 to 15 repetitions, 3 times per day.

In addition to Kegels, there are other exercises that can help strengthen the pelvic floor muscles, including:

1. Bridges: Lie on your back with your knees bent and feet flat on the floor. Lift your hips up off the floor, squeezing your glutes and pelvic floor muscles. Hold for 5 seconds, then lower back down. Repeat for 10 to 15 repetitions.

2. Squats: Stand with your feet shoulder-width apart and toes pointing forward. Lower your body down into a squat, keeping your back straight and your weight in your heels. As you stand back up, squeeze your glutes and pelvic floor muscles. Repeat for 10 to 15 repetitions.

3. Lunges: Stand with your feet hip-width apart and take a big step forward with your right foot. Lower your body down into a lunge, keeping your back straight and your weight in your heels. As you stand back up, squeeze your glutes and pelvic floor muscles. Repeat on the other side, and continue alternating for 10 to 15 repetitions.

By incorporating Kegels and other pelvic floor exercises into your daily routine during pregnancy and postpartum, you can help maintain good pelvic floor health and reduce the risk of complications such as incontinence or pelvic organ prolapse.

Integrating Pelvic Floor Exercises into Your Workouts

Integrating pelvic floor exercises into your workouts can help you maintain good pelvic floor health and prevent complications during and after pregnancy. Here are some tips on how to incorporate pelvic floor exercises into your workouts:

1. Start with Kegels: Kegels are a great place to start when it comes to pelvic floor exercises. They can be done anywhere, at any time, and don't require any equipment. Start by doing 10 to 15 repetitions, 3 times per day. Once you feel comfortable with this, you can start incorporating Kegels into your workouts.

2. Use the Breath: When doing pelvic floor exercises during your workouts, it's important to use the breath. Inhale deeply, then exhale as you contract the pelvic floor muscles. This can help you connect with the muscles and ensure that you're doing the exercises correctly.

3. Focus on Form: When doing exercises that target the pelvic floor, such as squats or lunges, it's important to focus on form. Make sure that you're engaging your pelvic floor muscles throughout the movement, and avoid bearing down or straining.

4. Progress Gradually: Just like with any other exercise, it's important to progress gradually when it comes to pelvic floor exercises. Start with basic exercises like Kegels and bridges, then gradually increase the difficulty level. Avoid over-exerting yourself, and listen to your body.

5. Seek Guidance: If you're not sure how to incorporate pelvic floor exercises into your workouts, or if you have any concerns about pelvic floor health, seek guidance from a healthcare professional or a certified prenatal/postnatal fitness specialist.

By integrating pelvic floor exercises into your workouts, you can help maintain good pelvic floor health and reduce the risk of complications during and after pregnancy. Start with the basics, focus on form, progress gradually, and seek guidance if needed.

CHAPTER 6

Nutrition and Hydration

Nutritional Requirements During Pregnancy

During pregnancy, it's important to pay attention to your nutritional needs to ensure that you and your baby are getting the necessary nutrients for healthy growth and development. Here are some key nutritional requirements during pregnancy:

1. Protein: Protein is essential for the growth and development of your baby's tissues. Good sources of protein include lean meats, poultry, fish, beans, lentils, tofu, and dairy products.

2. Folate: Folate is important for the development of the neural tube, which forms the baby's brain and spinal cord. Good sources of folate include leafy greens, citrus fruits, beans, and fortified cereals.

3. Iron: Iron is necessary for the production of hemoglobin, which carries oxygen to the baby's tissues. Good sources of iron include lean red meat, poultry, fish, beans, lentils, and fortified cereals.

4. Calcium: Calcium is important for the development of the baby's bones and teeth. Good sources of calcium include dairy products, leafy greens, and fortified juices.

5. Vitamin D: Vitamin D helps your body absorb calcium, which is important for bone health. Good sources of vitamin D include fortified dairy products and fatty fish.

6. Omega-3 fatty acids: Omega-3 fatty acids are important for the development of the baby's brain and eyes. Good sources of omega-3 fatty acids include fatty fish, such as salmon, as well as walnuts and flaxseed.

7. Water: Staying hydrated is important during pregnancy to help support healthy blood flow, prevent constipation, and regulate body temperature. Aim for at least 8-10 cups of water per day.

It's important to talk to your healthcare provider about your specific nutritional needs during pregnancy. They may recommend supplements, such as prenatal vitamins, to help ensure that you're getting all of the necessary nutrients for a healthy pregnancy.

Meal Planning and Snacking Tips

Meal planning and snacking can help you stay on track with your nutritional needs during pregnancy. Here are some tips to help you plan your meals and snacks:

1. Plan your meals and snacks ahead of time: Planning your meals and snacks ahead of time can help you make sure you're getting all the necessary nutrients. Try creating a weekly meal plan and grocery list to help you stay organized.

2. Eat small, frequent meals: Eating small, frequent meals throughout the day can help you maintain your energy levels and prevent nausea and heartburn.

3. Choose nutrient-dense foods: Focus on including foods that are high in nutrients, such as lean proteins, whole grains, fruits, and vegetables.

4. Don't skip breakfast: Breakfast is an important meal, especially during pregnancy. Try to include protein and whole grains in your breakfast to help keep you feeling full and energized throughout the morning.

5. Snack smart: Snacking can help keep you from getting too hungry between meals. Choose snacks that are high in protein and fiber, such as a piece of fruit with peanut butter or a handful of nuts.

6. Stay hydrated: Drink plenty of water throughout the day to help support healthy blood flow and prevent constipation.

7. Avoid processed foods: Processed foods can be high in sodium and unhealthy fats, which can be harmful during pregnancy. Try to choose whole, unprocessed foods whenever possible.

Remember to talk to your healthcare provider about your specific nutritional needs and any dietary restrictions you may have during pregnancy. They can provide you with personalized advice and guidance to help you stay healthy throughout your pregnancy.

Hydration Guidelines

Staying hydrated is important during pregnancy to help support healthy blood flow, prevent constipation, and regulate body temperature. Here are some hydration guidelines to help you stay on track:

1. Drink plenty of water: Aim for at least 8-10 cups of water per day. You may need more if you're exercising or if it's hot outside.

2. Avoid caffeine and sugary drinks: Caffeine can be dehydrating, and sugary drinks can be high in calories and contribute to weight gain. Try to limit your intake of these drinks.

3. Choose hydrating foods: Some foods can help you stay hydrated, such as fruits and vegetables with high

water content, like watermelon, cucumber, and strawberries.

4. Listen to your body: Pay attention to your thirst levels and drink water whenever you feel thirsty.

5. Consider a sports drink: If you're exercising for longer than an hour, a sports drink can help replace electrolytes lost through sweat.

6. Talk to your healthcare provider: If you have any medical conditions that affect your fluid balance, such as gestational diabetes or pre-eclampsia, talk to your healthcare provider about your specific hydration needs.

It's important to stay hydrated throughout your pregnancy to support the health and development of your baby. If you have any concerns about your hydration levels, talk to your healthcare provider for personalized advice and guidance.

CHAPTER 7

Self-Care and Stress Management

Importance of Self-Care During Pregnancy

Self-care during pregnancy is essential for maintaining physical and emotional health. Here are some reasons why self-care is important during pregnancy:

1. Reduce stress: Pregnancy can be a stressful time, and stress can have negative effects on both you and your baby. Practicing self-care activities like meditation, yoga, or taking a warm bath can help reduce stress levels.

2. Promote better sleep: Getting enough sleep is important during pregnancy, but it can be difficult with physical discomfort and anxiety. Self-care practices like a relaxing bedtime routine or practicing good sleep hygiene can help promote better sleep.

3. Boost self-esteem: Pregnancy can bring changes to your body that may affect your self-esteem. Practicing self-care activities like getting regular exercise, taking care of your skin, or getting a prenatal massage can help boost self-esteem and make you feel good about yourself.

4. Improve physical health: Taking care of your physical health during pregnancy is important for both you and your baby. Self-care activities like eating a healthy diet, staying hydrated, and getting regular exercise can help improve physical health.

5. Prepare for labor and delivery: Self-care activities like prenatal yoga, meditation, or practicing relaxation techniques can help prepare you for labor and delivery.

Remember that self-care is not selfish - it's essential for your overall health and well-being during pregnancy. Talk to your healthcare provider about self-care practices that are safe and appropriate for you.

Stress Management Techniques

Stress during pregnancy can negatively affect both the mother and the baby. Fortunately, there are many stress management techniques that can be used to help reduce stress levels. Here are some effective stress management techniques to consider:

1. Exercise: Regular exercise can help reduce stress levels by releasing endorphins and promoting relaxation. Low-impact exercises like prenatal yoga, swimming, and walking are generally safe during pregnancy.

2. Relaxation techniques: Practicing relaxation techniques like deep breathing, meditation, or progressive muscle relaxation can help reduce stress levels.

3. Support system: Having a strong support system can help reduce stress levels. Consider joining a prenatal support group or talking to friends and family members about your feelings.

4. Time management: Poor time management can increase stress levels. Consider making a to-do list or setting aside time for important tasks to help reduce stress levels.

5. Mindfulness: Practicing mindfulness involves being present at the moment and focusing on your thoughts and feelings without judgment. Mindfulness practices like yoga and meditation can help reduce stress levels.

6. Self-care: Taking care of yourself is important for reducing stress levels. Consider taking a warm bath, getting a prenatal massage, or indulging in a favorite hobby.

Remember, if you are experiencing excessive stress or anxiety during pregnancy, it's important to talk to your healthcare provider for support and guidance. They can help you determine which stress management techniques are safe and effective for you.

Getting Enough Rest and Sleep

Getting enough rest and sleep is essential for maintaining physical and emotional health during pregnancy. Here are some reasons why rest and sleep are important during pregnancy:

1. Reduce fatigue: Pregnancy can cause fatigue and exhaustion, especially in the first and third trimesters. Getting enough rest and sleep can help reduce fatigue and improve energy levels.

2. Promote healthy fetal development: Rest and sleep are important for healthy fetal development. During sleep, the body produces growth hormones that are necessary for fetal development.

3. Reduce the risk of complications: Lack of sleep has been linked to an increased risk of complications during pregnancy, such as preterm labor, gestational diabetes, and high blood pressure.

4. Improve mood: Getting enough rest and sleep can help improve mood and reduce the risk of depression and anxiety during pregnancy.

Here are some tips for getting enough rest and sleep during pregnancy:

1. Develop a bedtime routine: Developing a bedtime routine can help promote better sleep. Consider taking a warm bath, drinking chamomile tea, or practicing relaxation techniques before bed.

2. Create a comfortable sleeping environment: Create a comfortable sleeping environment by investing in a supportive mattress, comfortable pillows, and cool sheets.

3. Prioritize sleep: Prioritize sleep by making it a priority in your daily routine. Consider taking naps when possible and going to bed at a consistent time each night.

4. Avoid caffeine and stimulating activities before bed: Avoid caffeine and stimulating activities before bed, such as watching TV or using electronic devices, as these can interfere with sleep.

Remember, if you are experiencing difficulty sleeping or have concerns about your sleep patterns during pregnancy, it's important to talk to your healthcare provider for support and guidance. They can help you determine which sleep techniques are safe and effective for you.

CONCLUSION

Staying Active After Pregnancy

Staying active after pregnancy is important for physical and mental health. Exercise can help restore strength and energy levels, promote weight loss, and improve mood. Here are some tips for staying active after pregnancy:

1. Start slow: It's important to start slow and gradually increase the intensity and duration of exercise. This can help prevent injury and allow the body to adjust to physical activity.

2. Consider postpartum-specific exercise programs: There are specific exercise programs designed for postpartum women that focus on rebuilding core strength and pelvic floor muscles. These programs can be beneficial in restoring strength and preventing injury.

3.   Incorporate   strength   training: Incorporating strength training can help rebuild muscle strength and promote weight loss. Focus on exercises that target major muscle groups, such as squats, lunges, and push-ups.

4. Find time-efficient workouts: As a new mom, finding time for exercise can be challenging. Look for time-efficient workouts, such as high-intensity interval training (HIIT) or circuit training, that can be completed in 20-30 minutes.

5. Get outside: Getting outside and going for a walk or jog with your baby can be a great way to stay active and get fresh air. Just be sure to choose safe and appropriate outdoor activities based on your fitness level and recovery.

Remember, it's important to listen to your body and take things slow as you start to exercise after pregnancy. If you experience any pain or discomfort, it's important to stop and consult with your healthcare provider.

With time and patience, staying active after pregnancy can help promote physical and mental well-being.

Final Thoughts and Recommendations

Congratulations on taking the initiative to stay active and prioritize your health during pregnancy! Here are some final thoughts and recommendations to help you stay on track and achieve your fitness goals:

1. Listen to your body: Your body is going through a lot of changes during pregnancy, so it's important to listen to it and modify your exercise routine as needed. If something doesn't feel right, stop and consult with your healthcare provider.

2. Stay motivated: It's easy to lose motivation, especially as your pregnancy progresses. Try to stay motivated by setting achievable goals, tracking your progress, and finding a workout buddy or accountability partner.

3. Prioritize self-care: Taking care of yourself is just as important as taking care of your baby. Prioritize self-care by getting enough rest, eating well, and finding ways to manage stress.

4. Consult with your healthcare provider: Before starting any exercise program, it's important to consult with your healthcare provider to ensure it's safe for you and your baby. They can provide personalized recommendations and guidance based on your health status and pregnancy.

Remember, staying active during pregnancy can have a wide range of benefits for both you and your baby. By following the guidelines and recommendations in this book, you can safely and effectively incorporate exercise into your pregnancy journey and beyond. Best of luck on your fitness journey!